BASIC LIFE SUPPORT (BLS) PROVIDER MANUAL
A Comprehensive Guide
Covering the Latest Guidelines

M. Mastenbjörk M.D.
S. Meloni M.D.

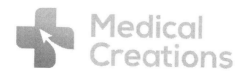

CONTENTS

YOU MIGHT ALSO NEED

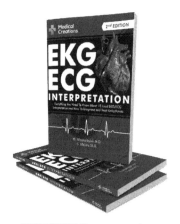

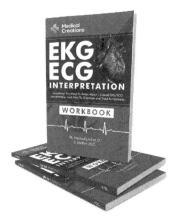

EKG/ECG Interpretation:
Everything you Need to Know about the 12 - Lead ECG/EKG Interpretation and How to Diagnose and Treat Arrhythmias (2nd Edition)

EKG/ECG Interpretation:
Everything you Need to Know about the 12 - Lead ECG/EKG Interpretation and How to Diagnose and Treat Arrhythmias: Workbook

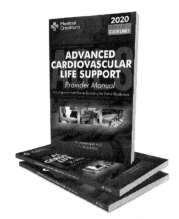

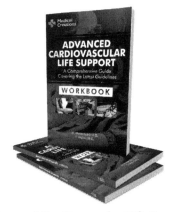

Advanced Cardiovascular Life Support:
Provider Manual - A Comprehensive Guide Covering the Latest Guidelines

Advanced Cardiovascular Life Support:
Provider Manual - A Comprehensive Guide Covering the Latest Guidelines: Workbook

Scan the QR Code

FREE GIFT

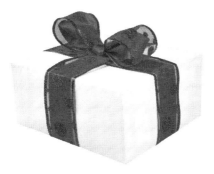

GET ONE OF THESE EBOOKS FOR FREE:

Medical Reference Pamphlet
ACLS ebook
Pulmonology ebook
Neurology ebook
Mini Medical Dictionary
Medical Terminology Digital Pamphlet
ECG Digital Reference Pamphlet

Scan the following QR Code:

You will be redirected to our website.
Follow the instructions to claim your free gift.

CHAPTER 1

Introduction to Basic Life Support

The ability to save a human life is an invaluable skill that can be of immense consequence. Therefore, it must be fostered at every possible opportunity. While it is not possible for everyone to undergo the years of training needed to become a doctor or a nurse, a basic knowledge of life-saving procedures can help make a difference in an emergency situation. Basic Life Support (BLS) refers to a set of procedures that can be learnt to prolong survival in life-threatening situations, until more professional help is available. Any individual can become certified in basic life support protocols. These protocols are frequently updated, based on the latest evidence available, and every individual who undergoes BLS certification may need to refresh their knowledge every two years.

Medical professionals usually have a sound understanding of basic life support protocols. Even then, it is essential for them to frequently undergo certifications to update their knowledge regarding the latest evidence-based protocols. This handbook is designed for both medical professionals and non-healthcare individuals. It aims to establish a sound understanding of the mechanisms underlying basic life support. The content in this handbook is in compliance with the 2020 guidelines recently released by the American Heart Association – therefore, all the protocols illustrated here are based on up-to-date evidence.

CHAPTER 2

Guidelines for Basic Life Support – A Review of the Most Recent Updates

Most organizations that offer training for Basic Life Support follow guidelines that are given by the American Heart Association. These are evidence-based guidelines, and as such, are reviewed every five years based on the scientific evidence available in literature. The latest version of their guidelines was released in October 2020. A short summary of the important changes is given below:

- Laypeople are encouraged to initiate early CPR. Early initiation plays a key role in survival. It is suggested that emergency medical teams use mobile technology to alert willing bystanders to perform CPR.

- The 'chain of survival' has been modified, with a sixth link, recovery, being added for both adults and children (refer to Unit V).

- For children, the rate for assisted ventilation has been modified. The current guidelines recommend delivery of one breath every 2 to 3 seconds, with 20 to 30 breaths per minute.

- Specific algorithms have been suggested for opioid-associated emergencies, for both adults and children. It is recommended that lay rescuers receive training in administering naloxone (refer to Unit VI).

- Emphasis has been placed on debriefing the rescuer – whether lay rescuers, emergency personnel, or hospital workers (refer to Unit VIII).

- The use of algorithms in training material and programs is encouraged, to enable easy recollection of protocols.

CHAPTER 3

Why Do We Need Basic Life Support?

Basic Life Support (BLS) is needed to sustain and prolong life till an individual can get proper, professional help. A large number of medical emergencies, such as cardiac arrests, occur outside hospitals. Getting access to immediate basic life support has been shown to increase survival rates and increase viable brain function. Before going on to how basic life support helps achieve this, we need to first understand basic life processes.

Understanding Life Processes: The Heart-Lung Cycle

Heart and lungs are the two key organs of the body that are essential to survival. Right side of the heart receives blood from rest of the body, and pumps it into the lungs. Lungs purify the blood by removing carbon dioxide and adding oxygen into the blood. The pure blood returns from the lungs to left side of the heart, which then pumps it to the rest of the body. The oxygen that blood delivers is essential for functioning of various parts of the body (Figure 1).

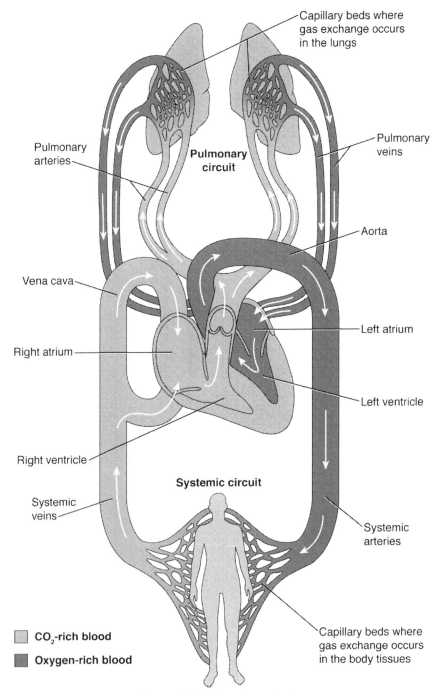

Capillary beds where gas exchange occurs in the lungs

Pulmonary arteries

Pulmonary circuit

Pulmonary veins

Aorta

Vena cava

Left atrium

Right atrium

Left ventricle

Right ventricle

Systemic circuit

Systemic veins

Systemic arteries

CO_2-rich blood

Oxygen-rich blood

Capillary beds where gas exchange occurs in the body tissues

Figure 1. The Heart-Lung Cycle

6

What are Life-Threatening Events?

Any event that causes an interruption of this basic heart-lung cycle has the potential to become a life-threatening event. There are three key life-threatening events:

Cardiac arrest: Cardiac arrest is defined as an abrupt cessation of heart function. This may or may not be preceded by other symptoms, and can occur due to several causes (Table1). Basically, in cardiac arrest, the heart stops beating. This means that ability to pump blood – both to the lungs, and to the rest of the body, is lost. The first organ to become affected by the lack of oxygen supply is the brain, and as a result, the patient loses consciousness.

If cardiac arrest is not reversed immediately, the continued lack of oxygen will eventually result in death. It is estimated that every year, 475,000 people in the United States die of cardiac arrest. Around 350,000 cardiac arrests yearly can occur out-of-hospital setting, where there is no immediate access to emergency care.

Table 1. Common Causes of Cardiac Arrest

CAUSES OF CARDIAC ARREST - 6Hs AND 5 Ts	
Hypovolemia	Tension pneumothorax
Hypoglycemia	Tamponade (cardiac)
Hypoxia	Thrombosis (pulmonary)
Hydrogen ion (acidosis)	Thrombosis (cardiac)
Hypo/Hyperkalemia	Toxins
Hypothermia	--

7

Respiratory arrest: Respiratory arrest is a condition where the lungs shut down, cutting off the ability to breathe. In most cases, this occurs after cardiac arrest, because blood fails to reach the lungs for the oxygenation process. However, sometimes, respiratory arrest can occur even when the heart is still functioning. This can occur due to nerve or neuromuscular disorders, and drugs that inhibit respiratory drive (e.g., Opioids). It can also occur secondary to trauma, which may produce a crush injury to chest or cause upper or lower airway obstruction.

Airway obstruction: This condition is closely related to respiratory arrest. While in respiratory arrest, the physiological act of breathing ceases, in airway obstruction, there is an anatomical (or physical) obstruction to the flow of air. This could be at any level from the nose, pharynx, larynx, or lower air passages.

How can Basic Life Support Help?

Basic Life Support attempts to stimulate the body to continue the heart-lung cycle. This is achieved through two key mechanisms:

- **Cardiopulmonary resuscitation (CPR):** This method aims at activating both the heart and the lungs. Heart is stimulated externally through chest compressions, while lungs are stimulated through rescue breathing. CPR involves a combination of both these procedures in a standard, regulated manner.

- **Relief of choking:** Choking blocks the upper airway, and cannot be relieved through CPR. Procedures that relieve choking basically attempt to dislodge the obstruction in the upper airway, and expel the obstruction through the mouth. Relief of choking is different from conventional CPR and is hence dealt with in a separate chapter.

The length of time that BLS must continue is still debatable. It has the capacity to sustain life as long as it is continued, but it is exhausting and the quality of support provided may deteriorate if the provider is not relieved within a set period of time. Practically speaking, if there is no spontaneous return of circulation (that is, the heart does not start to beat again on its own), advanced methods of life support must take over as soon as possible. These can only be provided by certified healthcare professionals. Therefore, before beginning BLS, or as soon as BLS is started, the rescuer must ensure that emergency medical services are being notified.

Time is of the Essence in Basic Life Support

Once a heart stops beating, there is a very small window period in which BLS can be performed to sustain life. When CPR is performed within the first two to three minutes after cardiac arrest, the chances of survival can triple. If CPR is delayed beyond this time, neuronal damage begins in the brain, which can lead to long-term loss of brain function, even if the patient does recover.

For this reason, most training organizations advocate specific algorithms that must be followed while administering BLS. Training centers offer several rounds of simulation using these algorithms, so that in a real emergency, the rescuer is immediately aware of what has to be performed, and does not hesitate. In the subsequent chapters, we will list algorithms that are in line with the most up-to-date guidelines released by professional organizations.

1. Which of the following is not immediately a life-threatening event?

   a. Cardiac arrest
   b. Heart attack
   c. Respiratory arrest
   d. Airway obstruction

2. Which of the following groups of individuals can administer Basic Life Support?

   a. Physicians
   b. Emergency Medical Responders
   c. Trained observers
   d. All of the above

3. Which of the following organs is irreversibly affected if CPR is delayed beyond three minutes?

   a. Kidney
   b. Liver
   c. Brain
   d. Lungs

CHAPTER 4

Breakdown of Techniques Used in Basic Life Support Algorithms

When training for Basic Life Support, you are expected to use a series of techniques in a regulated manner. Before practicing the exact algorithm, it is wise to learn all about each individual technique used in the algorithm. The next few units will focus on the components of cardiopulmonary resuscitation, including chest compressions, airway maintenance, and rescue breathing, and the use of an automated external defibrillator.

1. CHEST COMPRESSIONS

Chest compressions try to replicate pumping action of the heart from outside. The heart muscle acts like a sponge, and when the chest is compressed, blood within the heart is squeezed out into the major blood vessels. This blood cannot return back to the heart, because the exit of the heart (the junction between the heart and the major blood vessel) is equipped with tiny, one way doors called valves, which seal shut, and prevent backflow of blood. Once a few compressions are administered, the blood from the left side moves on to other parts of the body such as the brain, and the blood from the right side moves on to the lungs.

When blood flowing from chest compressions reaches the lungs, it may be oxygenated if the patient is also simultaneously receiving rescue breathing. However, it must be remembered that if an individual collapses from cardiac arrest, there already may be some oxygen left in the bloodstream. Therefore, the first priority is not to get oxygen into the blood; rather, it is to get the blood moving. This is why chest compressions always take precedence over rescue breathing in BLS algorithms. Current protocols place emphasis on 'hands-only CPR' if only one rescuer is present; this technique involves only chest compressions, without any rescue breathing.

Technique to Perform Chest Compressions:

- Stand or kneel by the side of the patient, bending slightly forward as comfortable.

- Place the heel of one hand (usually the non-dominant hand) firmly on the lower part of the breastbone (the xiphisternum).

- Place the heel of the other hand (usually the dominant hand) over the first hand (Figure 2)

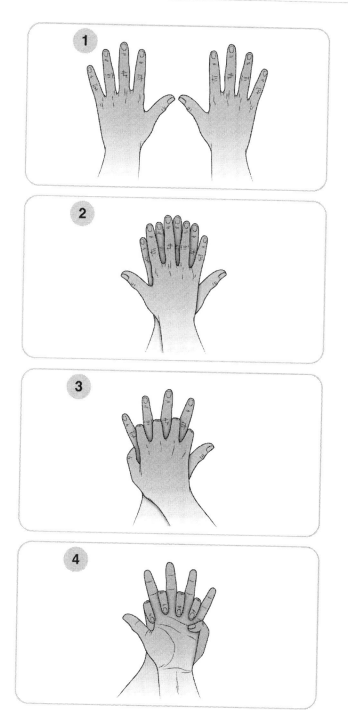

Figure 2. Correct Hand Positioning during CPR

- Ensure that your arms are straight, and position your shoulders directly over the heels of your hands, so that you are kneeling or standing 'over' the patient (figure 3).

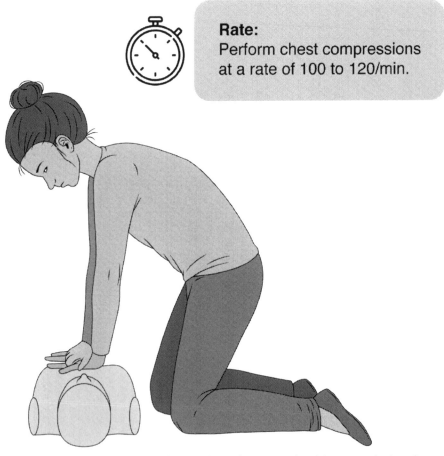

Rate:
Perform chest compressions at a rate of 100 to 120/min.

Figure 3. Extend your hands straight and position shoulders over the hands

- To give a compression, press directly down on the patient's breastbone, trying to achieve a depth of at least 5cm.

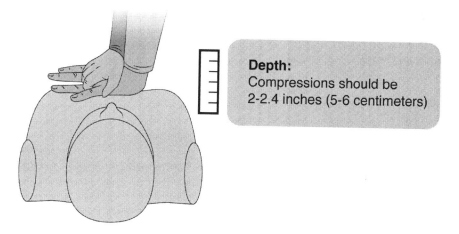

Figure 4. Depth of each compression

- Ensure that the chest recoils completely before you begin the next compression.

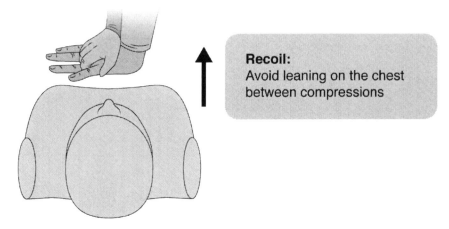

Recoil:
Avoid leaning on the chest
between compressions

Figure 5. The chest must recoil after each compression

- Aim to deliver at least 100 compressions per minute. The ideal rate is 100-120 compressions per minute.

Factors that Improve the Efficacy of Chest Compressions:

- **Depth:** For the heart to be squeezed adequately the depth of each compression must be at least 5cm. However, a depth of 6cm is likely to cause injury. Experts claim that most often, compressions are too shallow rather than too deep, so the focus must be on pressing down as deep as possible. If this is difficult to achieve, consider modifying the technique as follows:

  o As with the first technique, place the heel of the non-dominant hand on the breastbone.

  o Grab the wrist of your non-dominant hand with the other hand. When you compress the chest, supporting the wrist will provide added support and enable you to thrust deeper.

  o The modified technique is especially indicated if you suffer from arthritis or other joint conditions.

- **Recoil:** After each compression, the chest needs to recoil to its original position completely. This allows blood to flow back into the heart, which in turn can be squeezed out during the next compression. If recoil is incomplete, the heart is only filled partially, and this reduces the amount of blood that can be circulated during the next compression.

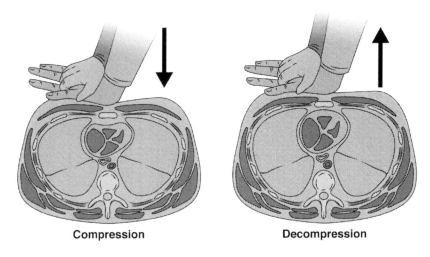

Compression   Decompression

Figure 6. Recoil allows the heart to fill with blood between each compression.

- **Surface:** It is essential that the patient be placed on a firm surface prior to beginning CPR. If the patient is lying on a soft surface, compressions can push the body into the surface, which reduces their efficacy.

- **Interruptions:** Adequate blood circulation is achieved only after several compressions are delivered. If there is any interruption in the delivery of chest compressions, the blood flow to vital organs, such as the brain decreases significantly. Once compressions resume, you will again need to deliver several compressions before adequate blood flow can be achieved. Therefore each interruption increases chances of neuronal damage and worsens the prognosis.

Chest compression must be practiced frequently on a dummy until the technique is perfected. After learning the technique, one can learn to integrate this into basic life support algorithms.

QUESTIONS

1. What is the minimum depth of a chest compression?

   a. 2 cm
   b. 4 cm
   c. 5 cm
   d. 6 cm

2. Why is recoil necessary between each compression?

   a. To give rest to the rescuer
   b. To prevent injury to the patient
   c. To allow the heart to fill with blood
   d. To allow blood delivery to the brain

3. How many chest compressions must be delivered per minute?

   a. 60
   b. 80
   c. 100
   d. 140

2. MANAGEMENT OF THE AIRWAY AND RESCUE BREATHING

Respiratory arrest may follow cardiac arrest, or may be an isolated event on its own. When a patient goes into respiratory arrest, two measures are taken to replace lung functioning – airway management and rescue breathing. In patients who have had cardiac arrest, current guidelines issued by the American Heart Association place more importance on chest compressions. If only a single rescuer is available, 'hands-only' CPR is advocated, which does not involve rescue breathing. Rescue breathing is carried out only under the following circumstances:

- When the patient is unresponsive, has a pulse, and is either gasping ineffectively or not breathing at all.

- In cardiac arrest patients after 13 minutes have passed or 400 compressions have been completed.

- When two rescuers are available on the scene immediately after cardiac arrest. One rescuer can focus on chest compressions while the other carries out rescue breathing.

AIRWAY MANAGEMENT

When a patient develops cardiac arrest, prior to delivery of rescue breathing, it is essential to ensure that the patient's airway is open and clear. Any obstruction to the airway (such as blood, vomitus, debris etc.) can impede air flow into the lungs and must be cleared using a gloved finger or a suction apparatus, if available. Larger obstructions that result in choking must be removed by specific maneuvers; these are discussed in detail in a subsequent chapter.

Apart from removing physical obstructions, the rescuer must ensure that the patient's airway remains as wide open as possible. This is achieved by any one of the following two maneuvers:

- Head Tilt – Chin Lift maneuver

- Jaw Thrust maneuver

- Head Tilt – Chin Lift maneuver (Figure 7):

    o Place one of your hands on the patient's forehead, and place the other hand beneath the chin, just under the bony part of the jaw.

    o With the first hand, tilt the patient's head backwards.

    o Simultaneously, use the other hand to lift the lower jaw and draw the chin forward. Ensure that you do not press too hard on the chin soft tissues; this might reflexively block the airway.

    o Ensure that the patient's mouth remains partially open so that rescue breaths can be effectively delivered.

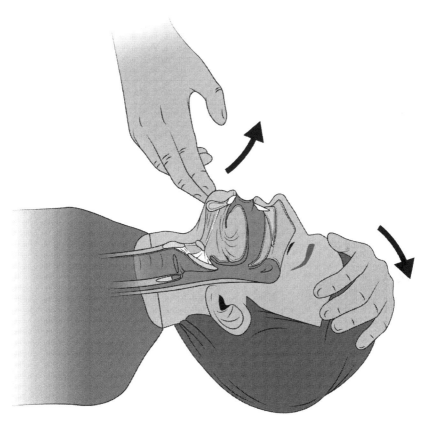

Figure 7. Head Tilt Chin Lift Technique

- Jaw Thrust maneuver (Figure 8):

    o This maneuver is preferred when the patient has a suspected head or neck injury. It avoids disturbing the cervical spine region.

    o To perform this maneuver, position yourself behind the patient. Rest your elbows on the firm surface on either side of the patient's head.

    o Position your fingers under the patient's lower jaw, just behind the angle of the jaw. Lift the jaw manually with both hands, so that the jaw is thrust forward.

    o As with the previous maneuver, ensure that the patient's mouth remains partially open.

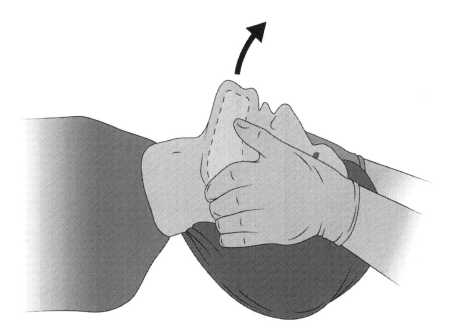

Figure 8. Jaw thrust technique

These maneuvers prevent the tongue from falling back and open up the airway, permitting unhindered air entry when rescue breathing is performed.

RESCUE BREATHING

Rescue breathing takes over the work of the lungs in the heart-lung cycle. The rescuer manually breathes air into the patient's lungs, which simulates the act of inhalation. This air helps oxygenate the blood flowing through the lungs.

You may wonder how rescue breathing works if you are essentially pushing 'impure air' into the patient's lungs. Yes, rescue breathing uses your exhaled air, which mostly consists of carbon dioxide. However, it also contains all the oxygen that your own body did not use, and this constitutes almost 17% of the exhaled air. This oxygen is enough to sustain life in the patient until better help takes over.

Use of Barrier Devices during Rescue Breathing

The most common form of rescue breathing is mouth-to-mouth resuscitation, which involves placing the rescuer's mouth over the patient's mouth. This places the rescuer at risk of coming in contact with the patient's body fluids. If the patient needing rescue is an unknown person, it is not possible to know if the patient has any communicable diseases that could potentially be transmitted while performing rescue breathing. Therefore, it may be advisable to use a barrier device to protect the rescuers from infection. Trained rescuers will usually carry a portable barrier device at all times. Two popularly used barrier devices are:

- **Face shield:** This is a flat, plastic sheet that can be placed over the patient's mouth and nose (Figure 9). It usually has a hole in the center through which air can be blown. The hole is fitted with a one-way valve or filter to prevent backflow of air and fluid. Face shields can be folded into small, tight packages that can easily be carried on a keychain. It is popular among non-healthcare workers who are trained in BLS.

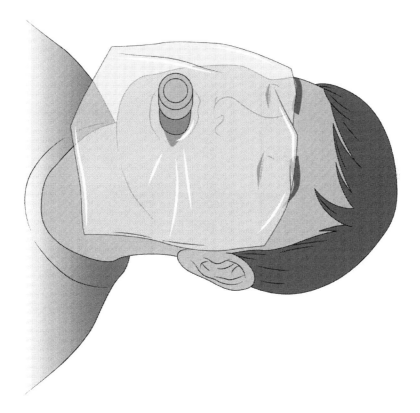

Figure 9. Face Shield

- **Pocket masks:** This is usually used by healthcare professionals and emergency responders. This is a pear-shaped mask which can be placed directly over the patient's nose and mouth to achieve a tight seal. In addition to a one-way valve, masks may have an oxygen inlet so that supplemental oxygen may be administered during the CPR procedure. The American Heart Association believes that these are more protective than face shields, and recommends replacing face shields with these at the earliest opportunity.

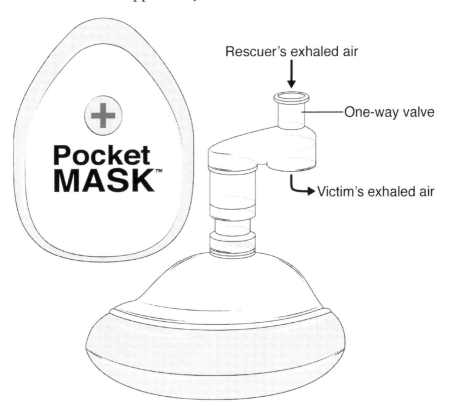

Figure 10. Pocket mask

What if no barrier devices are available? It is estimated that the odds of contracting a disease from the patient during CPR is 1:17,000,000. Therefore, if there is an urgent need for rescue breathing, the lack of barrier device should not stop bystanders from performing the same, even without a barrier.

Technique for Performing Rescue Breathing:

- Stand or kneel by the patient's side.

- Place the barrier device over the patient's mouth or nose, if available.

- Perform the head-tilt/chin-lift (or jaw thrust) maneuver to open the airway.

- Take a normal (not deep) breath.

- If barrier device is not available, pinch the nose closed with one hand, and place your mouth firmly on the patient's mouth, creating a tight seal (Figure 11).

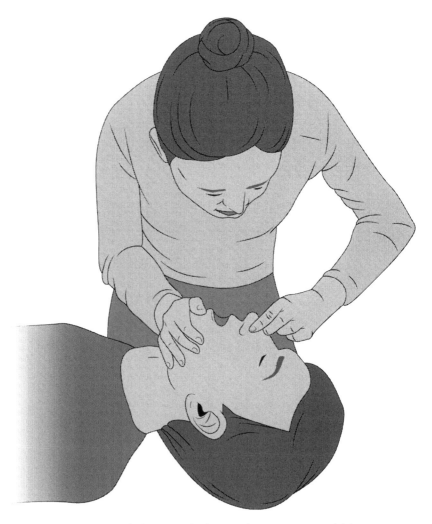

Figure 11. Pinch the nose if a barrier device is not available.

- Exhale into the victim's mouth, through the barrier device if available.

- The amount of air delivered and time taken to deliver the air must be monitored. Delivering too much air, or too fast, can force the air into the esophagus and stomach rather than the lungs. This increases the risk of gastric inflation. Ideally, ensure that each breath is delivered over 1 second.

- While delivering the breath, ensure that the patient's chest rises. This will indicate that the air is reaching the lungs.

- Repeat the procedure. Continue performing chest compressions if the chest does not rise even after two breaths.

- If you are administering rescue breathing to infants, mouth-to-mouth/nose technique is preferred. Your mouth should cover both the mouth and nose of the infant, creating a tight seal.

Ventilation using a Bag-Mask:

A bag-mask device (also known as an ambu-bag) is a device that delivers air under positive pressure into the lungs. If available, it must be preferred over mouth-to-mouth resuscitation. The bag-mask device delivers 21% oxygen, which is the normal oxygen level in room air. This is higher than 17% oxygen found in exhaled air and may be more beneficial to the patient. It can also be connected to an oxygen supply, which can deliver a higher percentage of oxygen. The technique for using the bag-mask device is as follows:

- The rescuer must stand at the head of the patient.

- Use the bridge of the patient's nose to guide the mask component of the device into correct position. Perform a head-tilt.

- Use the E-C clamp technique to hold the mask firmly in place, with your dominant hand.

- The thumb and index fingers of your dominant hand form a 'C', which is placed on the side of the mask, to press it into place and create a tight seal.

- The remaining three fingers form an 'E', which is used to lift the chin and open up the airway (Figure 12).

- Once the mask is firmly in place, use the non-dominant hand to squeeze the bag. The bag should be squeezed over one second, and with each squeeze, watch for the patient's chest to rise.

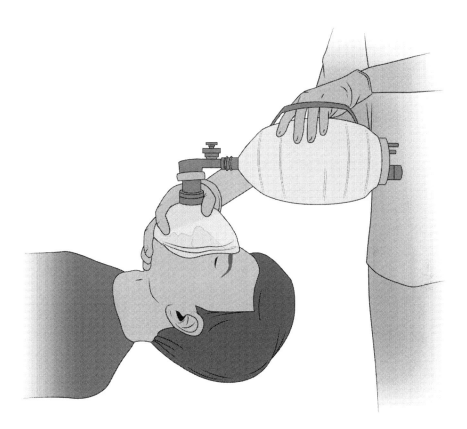

Figure 12. Use of bag-mask device. Note the E-C clamp technique used.

QUESTIONS

1. If a cervical spine injury is suspected, which of the following maneuvers can be used?

   a. Head tilt
   b. Chin lift
   c. Jaw thrust
   d. Roll over

2. Each rescue breath must be delivered over:

   a. One second
   b. Two seconds
   c. Three seconds
   d. Four seconds

3. If too much air is delivered during rescue breathing, what is the most likely complication?

   a. Lung collapse
   b. Gastric inflation
   c. Pneumothorax
   d. Brain injury

4. After how many minutes of 'hands-only' CPR must rescue breathing be started, if only a single rescuer is present?

   a. 9 minutes
   b. 11 minutes
   c. 13 minutes
   d. 15 minutes

3. Automated External Defibrillator - Why and How it is Used

Today, all CPR protocols involve the use of an automated external defibrillator (AED). This is a portable device designed for use by lay rescuers. This is used for patients in whom the underlying cause of cardiac arrest is abnormal heart rhythm.

The Need for a Defibrillator

Heart usually beats in a steady, regular rhythm. The rhythm of the heart is determined by electrical impulses that are spontaneously generated from a certain point in the upper heart, called the sino-atrial node. This electrical impulse spreads throughout the heart through a system of conducting fibers. Periodic generation and conduction of electrical impulses is essential for the heart to beat in an effective and steady manner.

Sometimes, there may be disturbances in either the generation or conduction of electrical impulses. These alter the rhythm of the heart. When the electrical impulses occur too fast, heart beat becomes fast and irregular. Fast, irregular heartbeats are referred to as arrhythmias. Two arrhythmias are particularly dangerous and are actually the leading causes of cardiac arrest. These are ventricular fibrillation and pulseless ventricular tachycardia.

- **Ventricular fibrillation:** There is disordered, electrical activity in the ventricles. As a result, the heart beat is completely unsynchronized and the heart begins to 'quiver' instead of pumping blood (Figure 13).

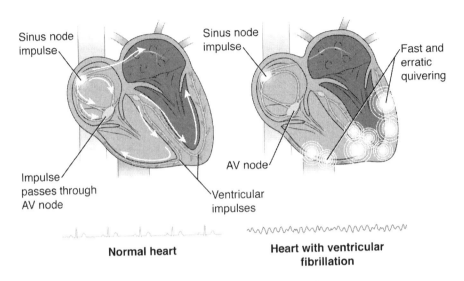

Figure 13. Heart in Ventricular Fibrillation

- **Pulseless ventricular tachycardia:** The ventricles begin contracting at an extremely fast pace. This results in inefficient pumping of blood. Due to the fast pace, a pulse cannot be felt.

When the above two rhythms are present, it is possible to 'shock' the heart into regaining its normal rhythm. In the hospital, this is achieved using a device called a defibrillator. It is important to note that only the above abnormal rhythms are 'shockable'. Asystole (complete loss of heartbeat) and pulseless electrical activity are also commonly encountered in cardiac arrest; however, these are not shockable. Therefore, prior to delivering a shock, through the defibrillator, the electric rhythm is assessed on a heart monitor and the healthcare worker needs to determine the kind of abnormal rhythm that is present.

AUTOMATED EXTERNAL DEFIBRILLATOR: DESIGNED FOR OUT-OF-HOSPITAL USE

As mentioned earlier in this book, a high percentage of cardiac arrests occur out-of-hospital. AED is a device that is designed for out-of-hospital use by individuals who have been trained in BLS. The device is lightweight and portable. Today, several places that witness gatherings of large number of people, such as shopping malls, airports, and amusement parks are equipped with AEDs. Of course, specific employees who work at such locations are trained in BLS and proper usage of the AED.

How the AED Works:

The AED is a battery-operated, computerized device. It consists of electrodes fixed on to adhesive patches, which are placed on the patient's body. These electrodes detect the heart rhythm and feed it into the computer, which analyses the kind of rhythm that is present. If the rhythm is shockable, the AED sends out a prompt to deliver an electric shock. The rescuer must then press the 'shock' button, which delivers a massive pulse of electrical energy through the adhesive pads. This 'shock' can stop the abnormal rhythm, and the heart resumes its normal function.

Most AEDs today are equipped with voice prompts. Once the rescuer turns on AED, the voice prompt issues instructions throughout the process, making it easier for even a lay person to operate the device. However, there are certain basic steps that are common to all AEDs, and these are described below.

Technique of Using an AED:

The AED is usually brought to the scene by another person, so it is assumed that one person is already performing chest compressions. These compressions must not be interrupted unless the rescuer is prompted to 'clear'. The steps detailed below must be carried out by the second rescuer on the scene.

- Remove the AED from its carry case and turn the power on. Some devices will power on automatically.

- Identify the correct adhesive AED pads to be used. Usually, adult pads must be used for patients greater than 8 years of age. You may need to peel the adhesive backing off the pads prior to attaching them to the patient's body.

- Place the adhesive pads according to the instructions issued by the voice prompt, and/or the diagrams given on the adhesive pads. Some common placement options are:

  o Anterolateral placement (Figure 14): One pad is placed on the front of the chest, directly below the right collarbone. The other pad is placed on the side of the chest, 7 to 8 cm below the armpit. This is usually just below and beside the left nipple.

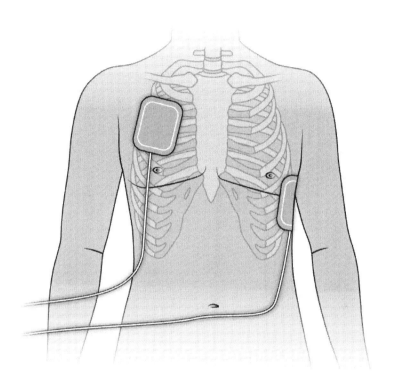

Figure 14. Anterolateral placement

o Anteroposterior placement (Figure 15): One pad is placed on the chest front. This is just beside the breastbone, below the left nipple. The other pad is placed at the back of the body, next to the spine on the left side. This placement is not generally preferred as it necessitates rolling the patient to place the pads.

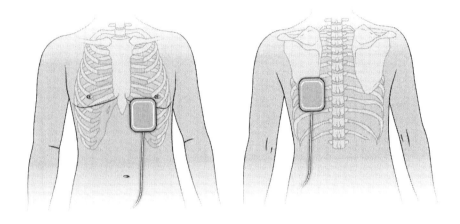

Figure 15. Anteroposterior placement

- 'Clear' the patient so that the AED can analyse the rhythm. While this may be an automatic process, some devices may require a button to be pushed for rhythm analysis.

- If the AED prompts to shock the patient, ensure once again that the patient is 'clear', and that no one is in contact with the victim.

- Press the required button to deliver the shock, if indicated.

- Immediately resume CPR.

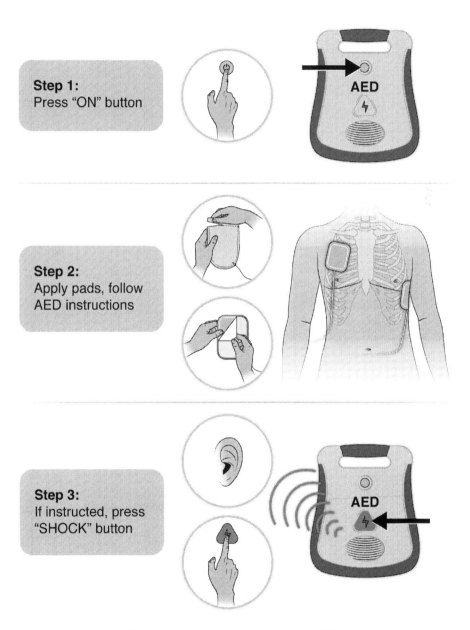

Step 1:
Press "ON" button

Step 2:
Apply pads, follow
AED instructions

Step 3:
If instructed, press
"SHOCK" button

Figure 16. Simple steps in using an AED

Factors to Consider while Using an AED

- Water: If the victim is wet, or has been lying in snow or water, it is important to ensure that the chest is wiped dry before using the AED. Water is a good conductor of electricity and may lead to electrical injury if not removed.

- Chest hair: If the patient has chest hair, the adhesive patches may not stick to the skin and the rhythm cannot be detected accurately. The chest hair must be shaved prior to applying adhesive patches. If a duplicate set of adhesive pads are present, it may be quicker to use the first set as a 'wax strip', that is, apply the pads and forcefully remove them so that the chest hair adheres to the pads and comes off. The second set of patches can be applied after this.

- Implantable pacemakers or defibrillators: Patients who have an existing history of cardiac disease may have undergone implantation of pacemakers or defibrillators. These devices may block the AED shock from reaching the heart. Such devices are easily palpable as hard masses beneath the skin. If present, avoid placing the AED directly over these devices.

- Transdermal patches: Several patients use transdermal patches for medications such as nitroglycerin, hormones, and nicotine. These patches may block delivery of electric current to the heart, and may also cause skin burns. If present, these patches must be removed, and the area must be wiped before adhesive pads are applied. The rescuer must wear protective gloves while removing such patches, or else there is a risk of the medication being transferred to the rescuer.

Time is of the Essence while Using an AED

If not normalized in time, both ventricular fibrillation and pulseless ventricular tachycardia can convert into complete asystole. Ideally, defibrillation must be provided within three to five minutes. Therefore, while it is imperative for a single rescuer to begin chest compressions immediately, the rescuer should also shout for help and ask for an AED along with a call for emergency medical services. As AEDs are readily available in many public places, it can be brought to the rescuer even before emergency medical help arrives.

―――――――――――――― QUESTIONS ――――――――――――――

1. Which of the following rhythms can be shocked by an automated external defibrillator?

   a. Ventricular fibrillation
   b. Atrial fibrillation
   c. Asystole
   d. Pulseless electrical activity

2. If the patient has an implantable pacemaker, which of the following is the most appropriate action?

   a. Do not use the AED
   b. Place the AED pads directly on the pacemaker
   c. Place the AED pads away from the pacemaker
   d. Use a magnet to divert energy from the pacemaker

3. What is the ideal time window for defibrillation to be provided?

   a. 5 minutes
   b. 6 minutes
   c. 8 minutes
   d. 10 minutes

4. TECHNIQUE MODIFICATIONS FOR SPECIAL CATEGORIES

In this section, we outline the modifications that are needed when basic life support is performed on specific categories of patients.

CHEST COMPRESSIONS IN INFANTS AND CHILDREN:

Chest Compressions in Children:

For small children, regular two-handed chest compressions may deliver too much force. One handed compressions may instead be used (Figure 17). Ensure that you are able to achieve the required depth of 5 cm with single handed compressions. If this is not achieved, the rescuer may switch over to two handed compressions.

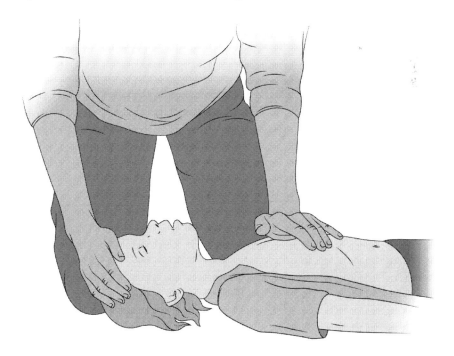

Figure 17. One handed CPR

Chest Compressions in Infants:

In infants, a single rescuer uses the 'two-finger' technique is used to deliver chest compressions, while two rescuers may use the 'two thumb encircling hands' technique.

For the 'two-finger' technique, the following steps must be followed (Figure 18):

- Use the index and middle fingers of your dominant hand

- Place the fingers on the lower part of the breastbone, just below the nipple line at the center of the chest.

- The depth of compression must be 4 cm, or around one-third of the infant's chest.

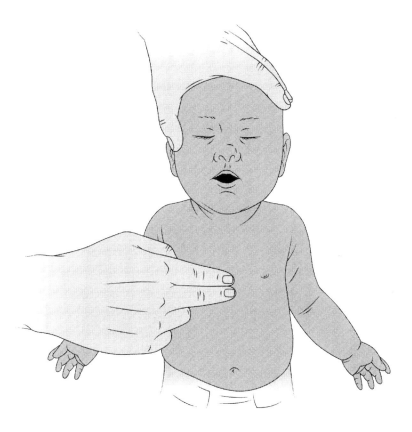

Figure 18. Two finger CPR

The 'two thumb encircling hands technique' is preferred to the above technique, because it provides better blood supply to the heart muscle, and can result in higher blood pressure. The depth and force of compressions is also more consistent using this method. However, it requires a two rescuer team, as the rescuer delivering compressions cannot easily disengage their hands to deliver rescue breathing. For the two thumb encircling hands technique, the following steps must be followed (Figure 19):

- Use both your hands to encircle the infant's chest. While the opposing thumbs rest on the infant's chest, the remaining four fingers of both hands are used to support the infant's back.

- The thumbs must lie on the lower half of the breastbone, just below the nipple line in the center of the chest.

- Use both thumbs to deliver chest compressions by depressing the breastbone. As with the previous technique, depress to one-third of the chest depth, or around 4 cm.

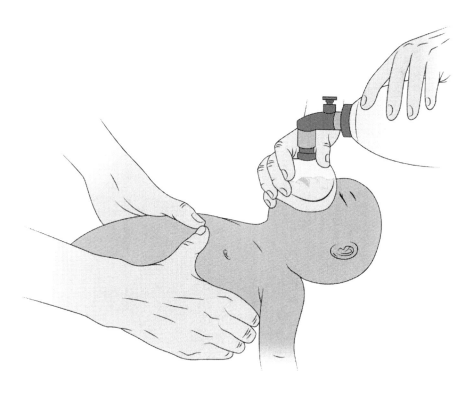

Figure 19. Two thumb encircling hands CPR

AIRWAY AND RESCUE BREATHING IN INFANTS AND CHILDREN:

The technique is almost the same as for adults, with a few modifications:

- In infants, the head-tilt must never exceed the neutral neck position. Excessive head tilt can cause airway compression (Figure 20). A good guide is the external ear canal, which must ideally be at the same level as the infant's shoulder.

- When using a pocket mask or a bag-mask device, ensure that the mask is small enough to fit snugly around the child or infant's nose and mouth. Several sizes are generally available in emergency kits, and the most appropriate size must be chosen.

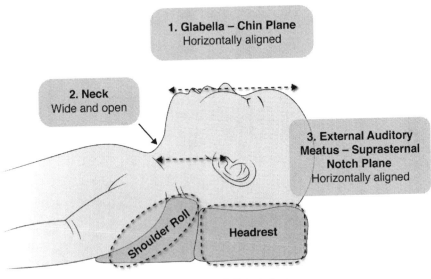

Figure 20. Head tilt in infants

AUTOMATED EXTERNAL DEFIBRILLATOR IN CHILDREN BELOW 8 YEARS OF AGE

While the shock delivered by a standard AED device is usually appropriate for patients above 8 years of age, it may be too high for younger children. For these patients, a reduced dose of shock must be delivered. AEDs may have one of the following modifications to make it suitable for children:

- A preprogramming option within the device

- A dose attenuator which limits the dose delivered by one-third

- Special pediatric cables

In addition to one of the above modifications, the AED may have special adhesive pads for children. For children, place one pad on right side of the chest above the breast. Place second pad on left side of the chest below the armpit. For infants, these pads are placed in anteroposterior alignment, on the upper left chest and back of the chest (Figure 21).

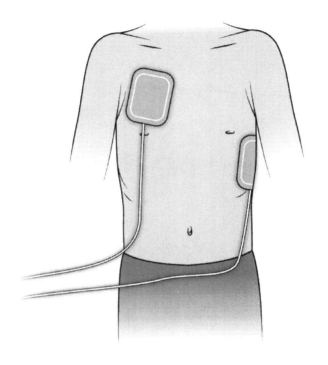

Figure 21. Anterolateral placement of child AED pads

For infants, if available, a manual defibrillator is preferred as the dose delivered may be adjusted manually. However, these needs to be operated by advanced personnel.

If a manual defibrillator is not available, an AED modified for pediatric dose may be used. For both infants and children below 8 years, if even this is not available, a standard AED may be used. *A higher dose of shock is preferable to no shock at all.*

QUESTIONS

---

1. Which CPR technique is the best for infants?

   a. One handed
   b. Two handed
   c. Two finger
   d. Two thumb encircling hands

2. What is the ideal depth of compression for infants?

   a. 2cm
   b. 3cm
   c. 4cm
   d. 5cm

3. What is the position for placement of child AED pads?

   a. Anterolateral
   b. Anteroposterior
   c. Posterolateral
   d. Mediolateral

CHAPTER 5

Protocols Used in Cardiopulmonary Resuscitation

Now that the individual components of cardiopulmonary resuscitation have been mastered, one must learn to fit these into an appropriate algorithm which can be followed when put into action.

Why is a specific protocol necessary for BLS?

Clinical protocols or guidelines are a set of instructions that must be followed when a healthcare intervention is carried out. Protocols and algorithms are always put together based on the best available evidence in the literature. Professional bodies usually review this evidence at regular intervals, and the protocols are then adjusted and updated accordingly. Because they are evidence-based, following set protocols can help optimize healthcare outcomes. When an evidence-based algorithm is followed for basic life support and cardiopulmonary resuscitation, chances of patient survival improve dramatically.

The concept of 'Chain of Survival'

The 'chain of survival' is basically a series of critical actions that, when followed correctly, can decrease the mortality associated with cardiac arrest. Each link in the chain is equally important in this regard. The chain of survival differs based on whether the cardiac arrest occurs in-hospital or out-of-hospital.

ALGORITHM 1: ADULT CHAIN OF SURVIVAL

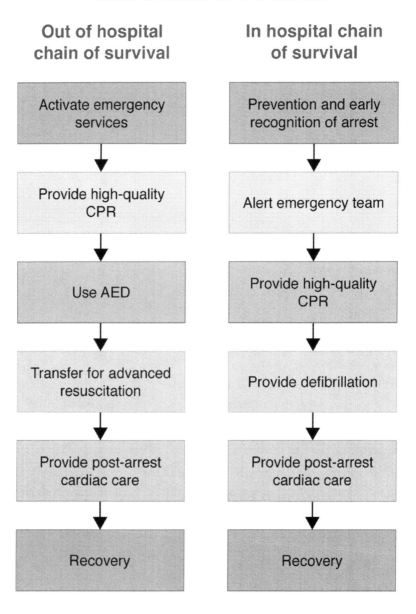

Out of hospital chain of survival	In hospital chain of survival
Activate emergency services	Prevention and early recognition of arrest
Provide high-quality CPR	Alert emergency team
Use AED	Provide high-quality CPR
Transfer for advanced resuscitation	Provide defibrillation
Provide post-arrest cardiac care	Provide post-arrest cardiac care
Recovery	Recovery

In this section, we describe the different protocols that must be followed for various clinical scenarios. The adult algorithm described in this section is based on the latest recommendations made by the American heart Association (AHA) in 2020.

56

ALGORITHM 2: ADULT BASIC LIFE SUPPORT ALGORITHM IN CARDIAC ARREST

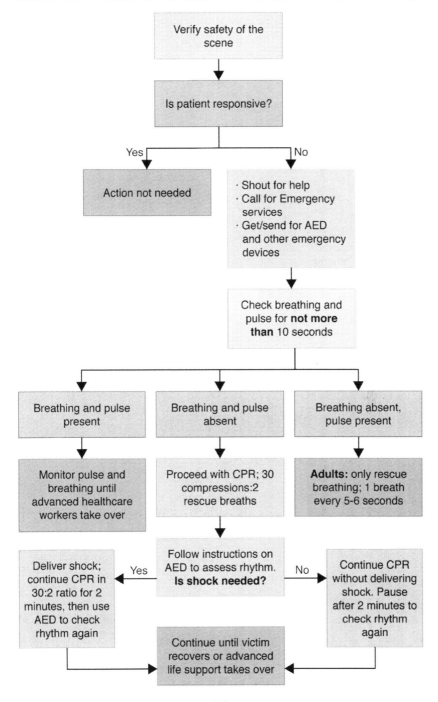

1. Basic Life Support for Adults

The protocol for BLS varies depending on the number of rescuers immediately available. A paramedical team will naturally have two or more rescuers available. If a lay person serves as a rescuer, however, it is likely that there may only be one trained rescuer on the scene. In each situation, the following basic algorithm must be followed.

ONE-RESCUER PROTOCOL

When only a single rescuer is available, the rescue protocol must follow the following phases:

Phase 1: Assessment of the external situation

- In the first phase, the rescuer must assess the situation in two parts – the environment and other people.

- Prior to attempting rescue, it is essential that the rescuer determines whether the environment is safe. For instance, in a fire or earthquake, the patient may need to be moved to a safer location where both the patient and rescuer are free from further harm. Rescuers must not put themselves in a situation where they may themselves become victims.

- After checking for responsiveness, if the patient is found unresponsive, the rescuer must call for available help. If other trained rescuers are present, the two-rescuer protocol may be followed (see below). If not, ask any untrained bystanders to activate emergency services and bring an AED.

If the rescuer finds himself completely alone, emergency services should probably be accessed through a mobile device prior to beginning CPR. The number for emergency services varies by country (For instance, it is 911 in the United States and 999 in United Kingdom). Trained rescuers must familiarize themselves with the emergency number used in their geographical location.

Phase 2: Assessment of the patient

- Briefly check if the patient is breathing (by looking for the rise and fall of the chest). This must be done in the shortest time possible and must not exceed 10 seconds. Gasps do not count as breathing. On the contrary, they may be a sign of developing cardiac arrest.

- Simultaneously, feel for a carotid pulse. To palpate the carotid pulse, feel for the patient's trachea with your fingers. Insert your fingers into the groove on one side of the trachea, between the trachea and neck muscles. As with breathing, *do not feel for more than 10 seconds.*

- According to the 2020 guidelines released by the AHA, the risk of harm due to CPR in a patient who is not in cardiac arrest is far less than the risk of delaying CPR in an actual case of cardiac arrest. Therefore, it may be better to proceed with CPR in a case of presumed cardiac arrest, rather than wasting time on assessing pulse and respiration.

Phase 3: Definitive rescue phase

The next steps will depend on whether breathing and pulse can be detected.

If the patient is breathing and a pulse can be detected:

- Monitor the breathing and pulse periodically, and check for responsiveness at intervals. This must be continued till emergency services arrive and the patient is given professional care.

If a pulse is definitely detected, but breathing is absent:

- Start providing rescue breaths. Deliver one breath over 1 second, every 5 to 6 seconds, totalling about 10 to 12 breaths per minute.

- Continue to monitor the pulse every two minutes. If the pulse cannot be detected, begin chest compressions immediately, as detailed in the next section.

- If an opioid overdose is suspected, a separate algorithm must be followed. This is detailed in a subsequent section.

If both pulse and respiration are absent:

- Immediately start delivering chest compressions. If possible, remove the clothing prior to beginning chest compressions. This improves efficacy of the compressions, and makes it easier to attach adhesive pads of the AED when it is made available.

- Deliver 30 chest compressions, followed by 2 rescue breaths. Continue this process in cycles of 30:2 compressions and rescue breaths, till an AED is made available.

- Once an AED is brought, it is assumed that the rescue scenario shifts to the two-rescuer process.

TWO-RESCUER PROTOCOL

If two rescuers are present from the beginning, the rescue process becomes more efficient. The rescue protocol will follow the following phases:

Phase 1: Assessment of the external situation

- When two or more rescuers are present, one rescuer must imediately take charge of assigning tasks so that the rescue process runs smoothly and efficiently.

- While one rescuer assesses the environment for safety, the other rescuer may be sent to activate emergency services and procure an AED.

Phase 2: Assessment of the patient

The steps in this phase are similar to the one-rescuer protocol.

Phase 3: Definitive rescue phase

- When breathing and pulse are both present, or pulse is present but breathing is absent, the protocol to be followed is the same as a single-rescuer protocol. If both pulse and respiration are absent, the two-rescuer team can work more efficiently.

- One rescuer starts delivering chest compressions, in a 30:2 ratio. Chest compressions must be delivered at a rate of 100 to 120 per minute.

- The other rescuer starts delivering rescue breaths at the rate of 10 to 12 breaths per minute.

- Once the AED is available, the second rescuer can attach the adhesive pads and allow the AED to analyze the rhythm. When the rhythm is being assessed, both rescuers must stand clear of the patient.

- If prompted, the second rescuer must shock the patient (while others stay clear). And immediately resume chest compressions.

- Delivering continuous chest compressions can cause rescuer fatigue, which may in turn decrease the efficiency of compressions, therefore, after every five cycles (or two minutes), the rescuers may switch places. This switch must be as quick and as efficient as possible, preferably within five seconds. The time taken by the AED to analyze the rhythm is a good time to switch positions.

- A repeat analysis of the heart rhythm must be performed every two minutes. The AED will usually issue a voice prompt to do so, and the rescuers may stop and switch over again at this point.

- This cycle continues until the patient recovers, or advanced life support providers take over care of the patient.

- Success of the two-rescuer protocol depends on effective communication between both members of the team. Chest compressions must be counted out loud, so that the other rescuer can correctly deliver rescue breaths at the end of 30 compressions. Clear communication is also essential while operating the AED, and instructions to stand clear of the patient during rhythm analysis and shock must be given in a loud, clear voice.

2. BASIC LIFE SUPPORT FOR INFANTS AND CHILDREN

Patients less than one year of age are considered infants, while patients between one to eight years of age are considered children.

Chain of survival in children:

In children, usually the underlying condition triggering arrest is not the heart. In most cases, children have trouble breathing, which in turn leads to arrest. Thefore more emphasis is placed on rescue breathing, and preventing arrest before it can occur.

ALGORITHM 3: PEDIATRIC CHAIN OF SURVIVAL

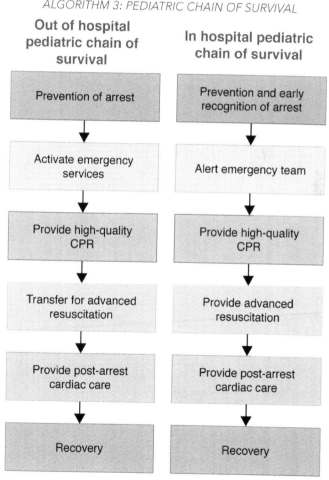

ONE-RESCUER PROTOCOL

The algorithm to be followed for pediatric collapse is outlined below:

ALGORITHM 4: PEDIATRIC CARDIAC ARREST ALGORITHM

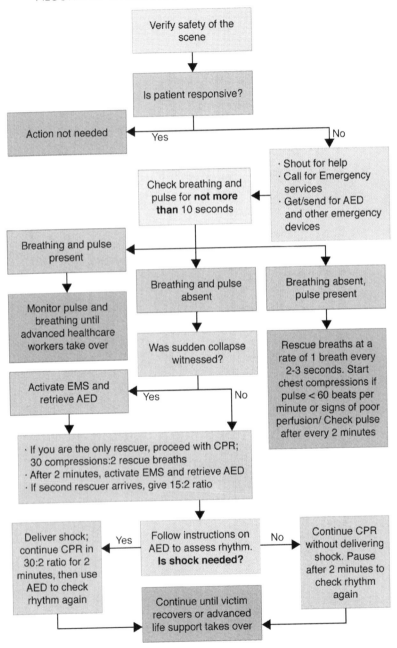

Phase 1: Assessment of the situation

- As for adults, the safety of the external environment must be assessed. Call for help, and activate emergency services as appropriate.

- Check for responsiveness by tapping the child's shoulder. For infants, tapping the heel of the foot may be done to check for responsiveness.

Phase 2: Assessment of the patient

Assessment of breathing remains the same as for adults. However, the carotid pulse may not be felt easily in infants and some children. For infants, the brachial pulse may be assessed, by placing two fingers in the brachial groove. For older children, the femoral pulse may be palpated by placing the fingers in the inguinal groove, between the hip bone and the pubic bone.

Phase 3 : Definitive rescue phase

If the patient is breathing and a pulse can be detected:

Similar to adults, monitor the child or infant by continuing to check on pulse and respiration.

If a pulse is definitely detected, but breathing is absent:

- Provide rescue breathing. Deliver rescue breaths over 1 second, every 2 to 3 seconds, totalling about 20 to 30 breaths per minute.

- Assess the pulse and perfusion. You may need to start chest compressions if:

- The pulse falls below 60 beats per minute.

- There are signs of poor perfusion, including pale or mottled skin, cyanosis, cool extremities, and weak pulse.

- If compressions are not necessary, continue with rescue breathing and check the pulse rate every two minutes. If the pulse falls below 60 beats, or is absent, start chest compressions immediately.

If both pulse and respiration are absent:

- The AHA advises two different recommendations based on whether the arrest was witnessed or not.

  o If the arrest was witnessed, the AHA recommends that you leave the victim to activate emergency services and locate an AED. CPR may be performed immediately on returning.

  o If the arrest was not witnessed, do not leave the victim. Instead, begin CPR immediately.

- Remove the patient's clothing to improve the efficiency of CPR and facilitate AED pad placement.

- Deliver chest compressions using 1 or 2 hand technique for children, and finger technique for infants. Compressions must be delivered at the rate of 100 to 120 per minute. The compression:ventilation ratio is 30:2. (30 compressions followed by 2 rescue breaths).

- After two minutes, if not already done, leave the victim to activate emergency services and obtain an AED. For children, it is essential that the AED be used as soon as possible. Use the AED to assess the rhythm and deliver shock, if needed. Resume CPR immediately.

- Reassess AED rhythm after two minutes, and continue the above cycle until advanced life support teams take over, or until the patient recovers.

TWO-RESCUER PROTOCOL

Phase 1: One rescuer takes the lead to assess the situation and determine safety. The second rescuer goes to activate emergency services and procure an AED.

Phase 2: Same as single-rescuer protocol.

Phase 3:

If the patient is breathing and a pulse can be detected:

- Monitor the child or infant by continuing to check on pulse and respiration.

If a pulse is definitely detected, but breathing is absent:

- One rescuer provides rescue breathing. The other rescuer assesses the pulse and perfusion. The second rescuer starts chest compressions if the pulse falls below 60 beats per minute, or there are signs of poor perfusion.

- If compressions are not necessary, continue with rescue breathing and check the pulse rate every two minutes. If the pulse falls below 60 beats, or is absent, start chest compressions immediately.

- The algorithm for ventilation alone is given below:

ALGORITHM 5: PEDIATRIC VENTILATION

Ensure correct head position	· **Head-tilt/Chin-lift maneuver** · **If neck injury: Jaw thrust**
Create a tight seal with mask	· **Use the E-C clamp technique to create proper seal**
Provide ventilation	· **Each breath over one second** · **One breath every 2-3 seconds** · **Do not over-ventilate**

If both pulse and respiration are absent:

- The first rescuer removes clothing and begins CPR using the two thumb-encircling hand technique (if infant), and 1 or 2 hand CPR (if the patient is a child). As soon as the second rescuer returns, he starts giving rescue breaths.

- For children, the compression-ventilation ratio is 15:2, if two rescuers are available. In children, rescue breathing plays a much more important role than in adults. This is because the cause of cardiac arrest in children is often shock or respiratory failure, which depletes the oxygen content in blood even before cardiac arrest occurs. Therefore, unlike adults, they do not have enough oxygen in their blood that can be circulated through compressions.

- As soon as the AED arrives, it must be used and shock delivered if needed. Rescuers can switch roles while the rhythm is being analyzed. Resume CPR immediately after shock (or after rhythm assessment if no shock is needed), using the 15:2 ratio. Reassess rhythm every two minutes, switching roles as needed.

- The above cycle must continue till advanced life support teams take over or the patient becomes responsive.

Table 2. Major differences in Adult and Child CPR

METHOD		ADULT	CHILD	INFANT
COMPRESSION: VENTILATION RATIO	SINGLE RESCUER	30:2	30:2	30:2
	TWO RESCUER	30:2	15:2	15:2
DEPTH OF COMPRESSION		5cm	5cm	4cm
VENTILATION RATE		1 breath every 5-6 seconds, 10 to 12 breaths per minute	1 breath every 2-3 seconds, 12 to 20 breaths per minute	1 breath every 2-3 seconds, 12 to 20 breaths per minute

QUESTIONS

1. Which of the following is not a sign of poor perfusion?

   a. Weak pulse
   b. Cyanosis
   c. Pale skin
   d. Warm extremities

2. Which of the following protocols uses a compression: ventilation ratio of 15:2?

   a. Single-rescuer for adults
   b. Two-rescuer for adults
   c. Two-rescuer for children
   d. Single-rescuer for children

3. How frequently must the AED rhythm be reassessed?

   a. One minute
   b. Two minutes
   c. Five minutes
   d. Seven minutes

CHAPTER 6

Management of Opioid-Associated Emergencies

The use of prescription as well as non-prescription opioids has increased considerably in the past few years. In 2017, the United States Department of Health and Human Services declared opioid misuse as a public health emergency and termed it the 'opioid epidemic'. Opioid overdose accounted for more than 232,000 deaths in the United States over the past decade. Opioids essentially cause central depression of the respiratory system, decreasing the drive to breathe. This can lead to respiratory and cardiac arrest.

Naloxone is a drug that serves as a specific antidote to opioids, and it can quickly reverse respiratory depression. If an opioid emergency is recognized early, administering this drug can greatly improve outcomes. Because of its serious, yet reversible nature, opioid emergencies are given special attention during basic life support training.

In their 2020 guidelines, the AHA outlined a specific protocol to be followed if an opioid overdose is suspected. The follwing algorithm is adapted based on their guidelines.

ALGORITHM 6: SUSPECTED OPIOID OVERDOSE IN ADULTS AND CHILDREN
- FOR LAY RESPONDERS

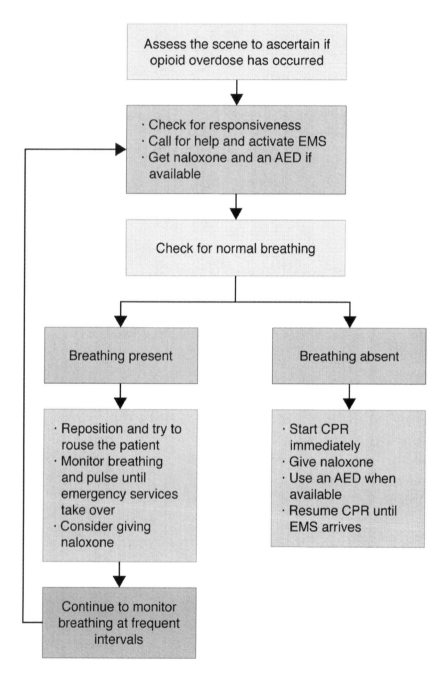

Assess the scene to ascertain if opioid overdose has occurred

- Check for responsiveness
- Call for help and activate EMS
- Get naloxone and an AED if available

Check for normal breathing

Breathing present

Breathing absent

- Reposition and try to rouse the patient
- Monitor breathing and pulse until emergency services take over
- Consider giving naloxone

- Start CPR immediately
- Give naloxone
- Use an AED when available
- Resume CPR until EMS arrives

Continue to monitor breathing at frequent intervals

How to identify opioid overdose?

- Ask the bystanders – they may have information on the patient's actions prior to collapse.

- Examine the scene for drug receptacles such as syringes or bottles.

- Observe the patient – injection marks, especially on the forearm, may be a sign of drug abuse.

CPR for patients with suspected opioid overdose:

- Trained rescuers may perform both compressions and rescue breathing for adults.

- Untrained rescuers should perform hands-only CPR.

Opioid overdose in children:

- The opioid epidemic has affected even children causing around 65 deaths in 2018.

- The algorithm for managing opioid overdose in children is identical to adults.

- The only modification is the method of CPR that is carried out. For infants and children, both trained and untrained observers must alternate compressions with rescue breathing.

1. Which of the following is an antidote for opioid?

    a. Pethidine
    b. Naloxone
    c. Oxycodone
    d. Felypressin

2. Who should perform hands-only CPR?

    a. Untrained observers for adults
    b. Untrained observers for children
    c. Trained observers for adults
    d. Trained observers for children

CHAPTER 7

Relief of Choking

Choking is the term used to describe the reaction that occurs when a person is unable to breathe properly because of a physical obstruction in their upper respiratory tract, usually at the level of the laryngeal inlet. In adults, the cause for obstruction is usually a piece of food. Children are more likely to swallow objects other than food, and foreign objects such as coins or small toys may also be responsible. Choking is a serious medical emergency. At least 4000 adults in the United States die each year due to choking. It is also one of the leading causes of death in children – it claims one child every five days in the United States alone.

Basic Life support training offers methods to recognize and relieve upper airway obstruction in patients. Adoption of appropriate techniques can relieve choking in 70 to 80% of all cases.

RECOGNITION OF A CHOKING VICTIM

A choking victim may not be immediately obvious to an untrained observer. However, prompt recognition will ensure prompt management, which increases the chances of a successful outcome. Therefore, it is important for all individuals training in basic life support to familiarize themselves with the signs of choking.

Signs of Mild choking:

Patients with mild choking usually have partial airway obstruction, so while there may be some difficulty in breathing, air exchange does occur at the level of the lungs. Some signs of mild choking are:

- Continuous cough in an attempt to expel the object

- A prominent wheeze between coughs

Signs of Severe Choking:

In severe choking, there is complete airway obstruction and as a result, air exchange is minimal or completely absent. This results in the following signs and symptoms:

- Patient is unable to speak at all or cry

- There is weak cough or cough is absent

- High pitched noise may be produced while attempting to inhale

- Cyanosis due to insufficient oxygen exchange

- Universal choking sign: This is an instinctive reaction and is considered the classical sign of choking (Figure 22). The patient holds or clutches their throat with the thumb and fingers of one or both hands.

If immediate relief from choking is not obtained, the lack of air exchange depletes the oxygen in the patient's blood. This causes the oxygen-deprived brain to shut down, and the patient may eventually lose consciousness.

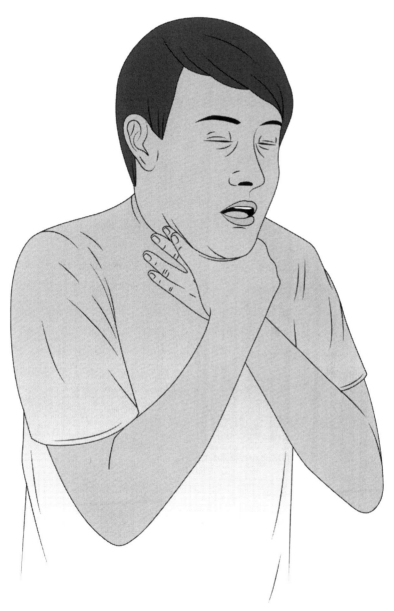

Figure 22. Universal choking sign

MANAGEMENT OF THE CHOKING PATIENT

Appropriate management of the choking patient depends on two main factors:

- Whether the patient is an adult, child, or infant

- Whether the patient is responsive (conscious) or unresponsive (unconscious)

RESPONSIVE ADULT OR CHILD: HEIMLICH MANEUVER:

The Heimlich maneuver (named after the physician who originally proposed the technique) is essentially a series of controlled, upward abdominal thrusts. These thrusts put pressure on the diaphragm, forcing it upwards into the chest cavity. This in turn pushes air out of the patient's lungs, forcing them to cough and eventually, expel the object. The Heimlich maneuver can only be used in a conscious person who is capable of standing or sitting upright. It is not intended for use on infants.

Steps in performing the Heimlich maneuver:

- Have the patient stand or sit erect.

- Position yourself behind the patient in such a way that you can wrap your hands around the patient's waist.

- Form a fist with your dominant hand. Place the fist, with the thumb side inwards, against the patient's abdomen. Your fist should lie in the midline, below the breast bone and slightly above the patient's navel (Figure 23).

- Use your non-dominant hand to grasp the fist of your dominant hand, and force it inwards and upwards, thereby delivering a thrust. The thrust must be oriented upwards, and must be quick but forceful.

- Repeat the thrusts until:

  o The foreign object is expelled and the choking is relieved; or;

  o The patient loses consciousness, in which an alternate method of management must be adopted. This is detailed in a subsequent section.

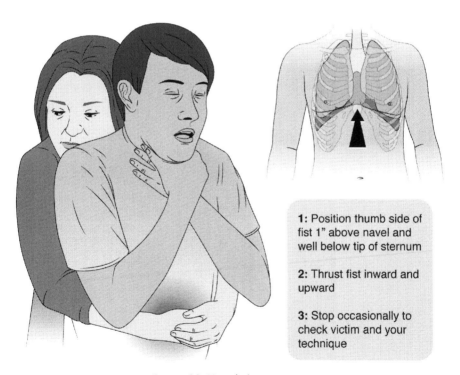

1: Position thumb side of fist 1" above navel and well below tip of sternum

2: Thrust fist inward and upward

3: Stop occasionally to check victim and your technique

Figure 23. Heimlich maneuver

MODIFICATIONS OF THE HEIMLICH MANEUVER:

Performing the maneuver on a pregnant patient:

It is not possible to perform abdominal thrusts when the patient is pregnant. Since the diaphragm of the pregnant patient is pushed upwards by the growing uterus, chest thrusts are performed instead of abdominal thrusts. Your hands should ideally be positioned at the base of the breastbone for this maneuver.

Combining abdominal thrusts with back blows:

While the American Heart Association recommends only abdominal thrusts for the responsive patient, other agencies, such as the Red Cross recommends a 'five and five approach'. To perform a back blow, like the Heimlich maneuver, the rescuer must stand behind the patient. Bend the patient over at the waist, placing your non-dominant arm across the patient's chest for support. Using the heel of your dominant hand, deliver a sharp blow right between the patient's shoulder blades. Alternate between five abdominal thrusts and five back blows, either until the foreign object is dislodged, or the patient loses consciousness.

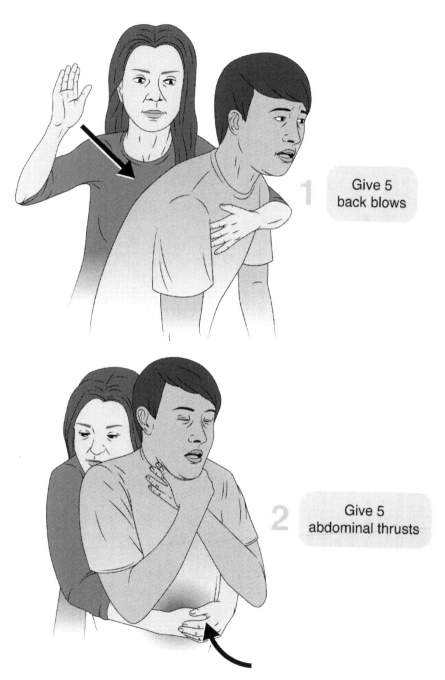

Give 5
back blows

Give 5
abdominal thrusts

Figure 24. Five and five approach

81

UNRESPONSIVE ADULT OR CHILD: CPR

When a patient loses consciousness, it is indicative of oxygen deprivation to the brain. Immediate steps must be taken to maintain circulation so that oxygen supply is restored to the vital organs of the body. The focus here is therefore on CPR.

The following steps must be followed when the rescuer is certain that the unconsciousness is the result of choking:

- Immediately call for help and ask any available people to activate the Emergency Response Services.

- Gently lower the victim to the ground or any available firm surface.

- Start performing CPR. As per the most recent guidelines, it is not necessary to look for a pulse – this may delay the resuscitation process. Perform 30 chest compressions, followed by two rescue breaths.

- Modification of rescue breathing: Before each cycle of rescue breathing, open the patient's mouth wide and look for the foreign object. If the object is visible and can easily be removed, the rescuer may attempt to retrieve the object. If the object cannot be retrieved, two rescue breaths may be given. DO NOT attempt to remove the object if it is not visible. A blind finger sweep may actually push the object deeper into the airway.

- Continue 5 cycles of 30 compressions and 2 rescue breaths. After 5 cycles, emergency services must be called for, if this has not already been done.

Continuing CPR after choking relief:

Chest compressions may function similar to abdominal thrusts and aid in dislodging the foreign object. With periodic inspection prior to rescue breathing, it may be possible to remove the foreign object and clear the airway. However, the patient may not regain consciousness immediately. The CPR must continue until the pulse and respiration recovers completely, or till the patient may be shifted to the hospital.

RELIEF OF CHOKING IN A RESPONSIVE INFANT

Abdominal thrusts must never be used in an infant. Instead, standard chest compressions, similar to those described for infant CPR, are used. The American Heart Association recommends the 'five and five' approach for responsive infants, however, the method is slightly different. The following steps must be followed:

- Sit on a chair, or kneel, holding the infant on your lap. If it can be done quickly, the dress must be removed – chest thrusts may be more effective when performed on the bare chest.

- For the back blows, hold the infant face down, lying on your forearm. Your forearm must be supported on your lap or thigh. Ensure that the head is at a slightly lower level than the chest, and use the palm of your hand to support the infant's head and chin (Figure 25). Ensure that your fingers do not compress the throat soft tissues, as this may obstruct the airway further.

- Using the heel of your other hand, deliver five back slaps between the infant's shoulder blades.

- To perform chest thrusts, turn the infant over from one hand to the other, in a single movement so that the infant now rests face up, on your other forearm. Rest the forearm on your thigh and ensure that the head remains lower than the chest (Figure 26).

- Perform five chest thrusts with the fingers of the other hand, using the technique described in the previous section.

- Continue alternating between five back blows and five chest thrusts, until the object is dislodged or the patient loses consciousness.

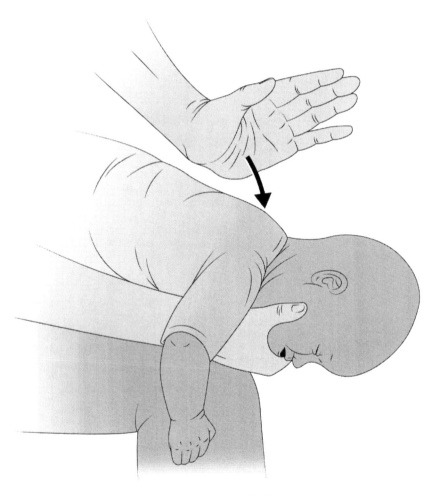

Figure 25. Supporting a choking infant

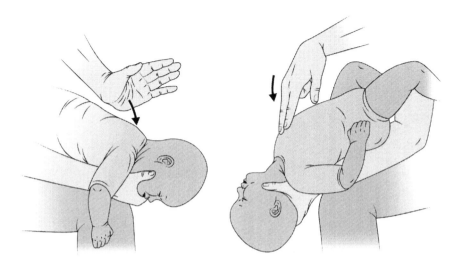

Figure 26. Choking relief for infants

RELIEF OF CHOKING IN AN UNRESPONSIVE INFANT

If the infant becomes unresponsive, the rescuer must shift over to CPR. As for adults, one must not waste time looking for a pulse. The following steps must be followed:

- Call for help and ask any bystanders to activate emergency services.

- Place the patient on a firm surface and start chest thrusts. Alternate between chest thrusts and rescue breathing.

- As for adults, before beginning each rescue breath, visually inspect the airway for the foreign object and attempt to retrieve it if it can be easily done.

- Call for emergency services at the end of two minutes, if it has not already been done.

--------------------- QUESTIONS ---------------------

1. Which of the following indicates mild choking?

    a. High pitched noise
    b. Continuous cough
    c. Inability to cry
    d. Cyanosis

2. Heimlich maneuver is not suitable for

    a. Adults
    b. Pregnant women
    c. Children
    d. Infants

3. How many back blows must alternate with chest or abdominal thrusts for choking relief?

    a. Four
    b. Five
    c. Three
    d. Six

CHAPTER 8

Conclusion: Post-CPR Care

Most rescuers are well-trained in the basic life support process at the end of a training course. However, because this is merely a simulator for real-life situations, often the rescuer finds himself at a loose end after the rescue operations are over.

When to stop CPR?

CPR must only be stopped by rescuers if any one of the following end points is reached:

- An advanced life support team takes over chest compressions and rescue breathing, while transporting the patient to the hospital.

- The patient begins to regain consciousness and awareness.

- The rescuer becomes fatigued to an extent that their own health may be at risk if they continue. If this is the case, there would usually be other rescuers on hand to take over.

Debriefing programs for the rescuer

- In their 2020 recommendations, the AHA recognized the fact that rescuers may themselves experience some anxiety or post-traumatic stress after the rescue operation is complete. With this in mind they recommend that:

- For trained teams, a debriefing must take place, to review performance and recognize stressors. Lay rescuers may also receive a debriefing, along with a referral for emotional support.

Answers to Exercises

CHAPTER 2

1. B
2. D
3. C

CHAPTER 3

Section 1 Chest Compressions

1. C
2. C
3. C

Section 2 Airway maintenance and Rescue breathing

1. C
2. A
3. B
4. C

Section 3 Automated External defibrillator - why and how it is used

1. A
2. C
3. C

Section 4 Technique modifications for special categories

1. D
2. C
3. A

CHAPTER 5

1. D
2. C
3. B

CHAPTER 6

1. B
2. A

CHAPTER 7

1. B
2. D
3. B

Index

JOIN OUR COMMUNITY

Medical Creations® is an educational company focused on providing study tools for Healthcare students.

You can find all of our products at this link:

www.medicalcreations.net

If you have any questions or concerns please contact us:

hello@medicalcreations.net

We want to be as close as possible to our customers, that's why we are active on all the main Social Media platforms.

You can find us here:

Facebook   www.facebook.com/medicalcreations
Instagram   www.instagram.com/medicalcreationsofficial
Pinterest   www.pinterest.com/medicalcreations

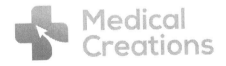

CHECK OUT OUR OTHER BOOKS

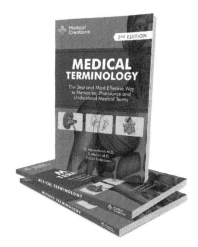

Medical Terminology:
The Best and Most Effective Way
to Memorize, Pronounce and
Understand Medical Terms
(2nd Edition)

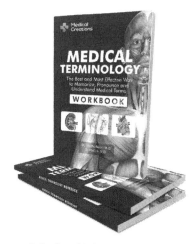

Medical Terminology:
The Best and Most Effective
Way to Memorize, Pronounce
and Understand Medical Terms:
Workbook

Scan the QR Code

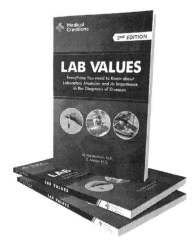

Lab Values:
Everything You Need to Know
about Laboratory Medicine and
its Importance in the Diagnosis
of Diseases

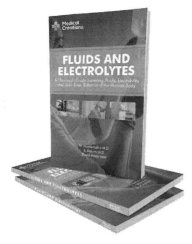

Fluids and Electrolytes:
A Torough Guide covering Fluids,
Electrolytes and Acid-Base Balance
of the Human Body

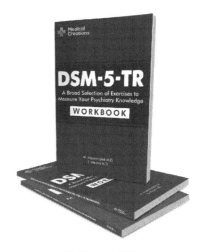

DSM-5-TR:
A Broad Selection of Exercises
to Measure Your Psychiatry
Knowledge: Workbook

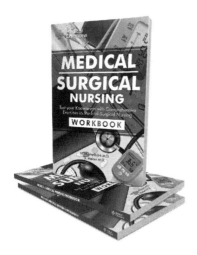

Medical Surgical Nursing:
Test your Knowledge with
Comprehensive Exercises in
Medical-Surgical Nursing:
Workbook

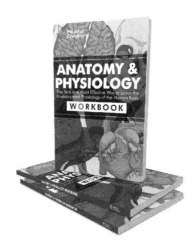

Anatomy & Physiology:
The Best and Most Effective Way
to Learn the Anatomy and
Physiology of the Human Body:
Workbook

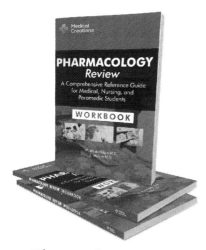

Pharmacology Review:
A Comprehensive Reference
Guide for Medical, Nursing, and
Paramedic Students: Workbook

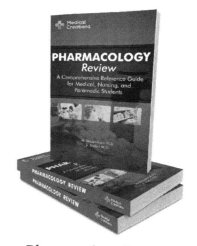

Pharmacology Review:
A Comprehensive Reference
Guide for Medical, Nursing,
and Paramedic Students

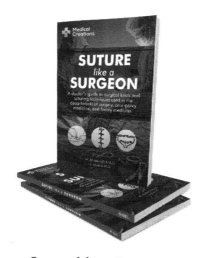

Suture like a Surgeon:
A Doctor's Guide to Surgical Knots
and Suturing Techniques used in the
Departments of Surgery, Emergency
Medicine, and Family Medicine

Medical Creations Suture Practice Kit with Suturing Video Series
by Board-Certified Surgeon and Ebook Training Guide

SUTURE LIKE A SURGEON PRACTICE KIT

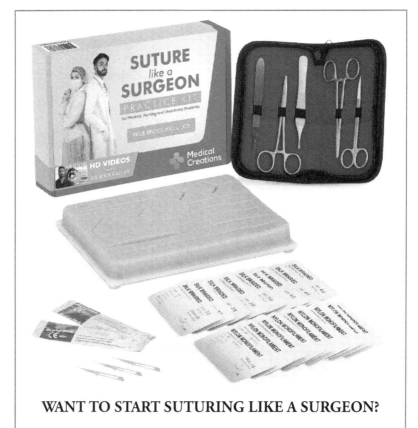

WANT TO START SUTURING LIKE A SURGEON?

Our Suture Practice Kit contains all of the tools
you need to start practicing.

Scan the QR Code

Made in the USA
Las Vegas, NV
05 October 2024

96343202R10057